# Her Little Soldier

### By Craig DeHut

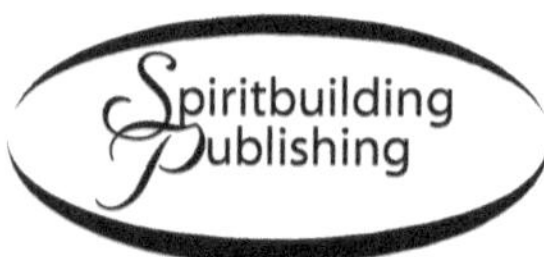

*Spiritual "equipment" for the contest of life.*

SPIRITBUILDING PUBLISHING
15591 N. State Rd. 9, Summitville, Indiana, 46070
*www.SpiritBuilding.com*

Dedicated to my mother,
for encouraging me, for believing in me,
and for never giving up.

# Table of Contents

# Introduction

I had condemned myself, but in a way I was glad.

"Heal them before you heal me," I would ask God in my prayers.

Whenever I heard of someone that was sick, it became my first instinct to ask God to heal them, without any thought of the sickness that I had.

When it finally dawned on me that God might very well be doing exactly what I had asked him to do, I cried. Mom held me in her arms and just let me cry. There were times that I thought I wasn't being strong enough, but what she told me that day would stay with me forever,

"You're such a little soldier, you know that?"

I didn't. I viewed myself as others typically did: a skinny, short, diabetic kid that hated looking at himself in the mirror because of the pale, sick looking figure that stared back. A soldier? Even with the wonderful imagination and creative mind that I had grown a reputation for, I never envisioned myself as such a hero.

I didn't, but my mother did.

It was that day that I started writing about my disease in my journal. At first they were simply short little blurbs at the beginning of each entry. They soon evolved into my fears, frustrations, and life lessons that came from having my disease.

I know that God is still healing others. I've decided to write this book in the hopes that I can share something with the world and continue to help God heal other people of their hurt.

I pray that my pain, my journey, and my discoveries may bring you some healing and inspire you. My desire is that you will never look at life in the same way again.

# Chapter 1
# My Story

My name is Craig Daniel Dehut. I like my middle name because every time that I hear it, I think of God's prophet in the Old Testament. Daniel was the kind of guy that, no matter what happened to him, never failed to believe in and stand for the one true God. Daniel, along with his friends, defied a king because they believed that no man was so great that he should be worshiped over God. They remained strong in hard times. I've always wished that I could be like Daniel and live up to my name.

I was ten years old when it happened. I was living with my father, Bruce, my mother, Linda, my four older brothers, Jeremy, Jeff, Darren, and Kurt and my younger sister, Lindsey. We were living in Bend, Oregon where my father was a preacher at our local congregation.

Bend is a mountain town in the area of Oregon called the High Desert. I was born in Salem, which is about a three-hour drive from Bend, down the mountain into the Willamette Valley. Because it was the place of my birth, we knew a lot of people around that area, so we traveled back and forth between Bend and the valley all of the time.

My older brothers were playing basketball with our homeschool sports league and we had gone down to the valley to attend one of their games. Before the game, I remember complaining that I didn't feel well. After looking back at photos taken from that day, I am shocked to see just how sickly looking I appeared. I was so pale and tired. We simply thought that I had one of those 24-hour flu bugs or something.

Right before the game, I spilled grape juice all over my shirt. Now, we're not talking about a little spot that I could cover up if I kept my arms crossed. It was *all* over my shirt. I told my mom that there was no way that I was going to the game with my shirt looking like it was, so my dear sweet mother, rushed to the nearest Wal-Mart store and grabbed me a cheap multicolored T-shirt so that I wouldn't have to be embarrassed at my brother's game. I must have been the luckiest kid alive at that point, to have a mom like her – and *it* hadn't even happened yet.

*Actually, it had already begun. We just didn't know it.*

Actually, it had already begun. We just didn't know it. The next morning we all piled into our cars and headed back home. Most of my siblings loaded into our huge, brown, 12-seater van, but my dad, my oldest brother Jeremy and I went in our yellow Chevy Luv pickup truck. When you talk about automobiles having character, this little truck had so much character that sometimes it seemed to talk to you through the gurgling of its engine. It was a great piece of machinery. That Chevy Luv never let us down.

We had only gone a little ways, when it hit me. I had to go to the bathroom and I had to go *bad!* We were fifteen minutes from the nearest town, but I knew beyond a doubt that there was no way that I was going to make it that long. Dad pulled the truck to the side of the road and I dashed out into the woods to relieve myself. A couple of minutes later, I was back in the truck and we were on our way again.

No more than thirty minutes went by and I was hit by the same undeniable urge. Believe me, I tried thinking about something else, but when you're driving through a mountain pass surrounded by waterfalls and rivers, it's next to impossible. My mind could not ignore what my body was telling it.

"We have *got* to pull over!"

I quickly darted out into the trees again, did my thing, and darted back to the truck. After that, I felt pretty good – for about another half hour.

I probably made three or four stops that trip. As we neared home, we pulled into a gas station and dad bought me a 7-up. My first swig made me realize that I was extremely thirsty. I finished it off within minutes.

When we got home, Mom made an appointment for me at

the Immediate Care center for the next morning. She figured that I probably just had an infection or something and that would explain why I had to go to the bathroom all of the time.

Even though that was what she told me, I could tell that she was still unsure about what was really wrong with me. I didn't ask any questions. I figured that I would go to the doctor the next day, he would take my temperature, make me swallow a pill, give me a sucker and send me home healthy and back to normal.

There was little chance that it was going to be that easy, and an even smaller chance that I would be going home with a sucker.

The next day, Mom and I went to the doctor. We sat together in the waiting room without saying a word. Mom just kept looking at me and holding my hand. That one moment is the one that has really stuck with me through these years. I remembering looking into her eyes and seeing how sad her heart was. It was almost as if she knew that it was more than a simple infection.

The doctor called us in and set me up on his examination table - the kind with that white paper on top that crinkles and makes a lot of noise when you move around on it. Mom told him my name and all of the regular information that doctors have to keep records of.

"What are his symptoms?" He asked.

My mother told him about how I had to use the restroom a lot. He wrote that down and kind of nodded his head. She also told him that I was really thirsty all of the time. He nodded his head again. I finally spoke up and asked him,

"Is it normal for me to be this skinny?"

He looked at me. I was ten years old and scarcely over seventy pounds. Something with the doctor clicked - he had heard this all before.

After a couple of quick tests, he took my mom out into the hallway and told her his diagnosis. She really didn't want to tell me there in that unfamiliar doctor's office. She asked if she could go home and get my dad so that they could tell me together. The doctor said that she couldn't and that she wasn't leaving that office until she told me. She came into the room and began to cry as she told me what was going on. I had been diagnosed as a Type

1 Juvenile Diabetic.

I had been cursed.

*Okay,* I thought, *so what pill do I have to take to make it go away?* My young, often naïve, mind didn't fully grasp the seriousness of the situation. It wasn't going to be that easy. He told us to go back home, pack a few things and get to the hospital as soon as we could.

I had no idea what was going on as Mom drove me home. Apparently, she had heard of this disease before and knew a little bit about it. At that point, I still didn't even know how to say the word, let alone what it meant to have it.

We walked into the house. Everybody else was sitting down watching a movie. It was *Mary Poppins*, I think. I grabbed some clothes while Mom explained to my siblings what was going on. My brother Jeff let me borrow his Gameboy to use while I was in the hospital. I was in and out and on my way to the hospital in less than ten minutes.

> *I can remember sitting in the hospital while another doctor told us about this mysterious disease called Diabetes.*

My memories about my trip to the hospital are few. I can remember sitting in the hospital while another doctor told us about this mysterious disease called Diabetes. The only things I really remember him saying were things like, "you can't eat sugary cereals like Cap'n Crunch anymore." My mom chuckled and said that I usually didn't eat those kinds of cereals anyway.

The doctors and nurses did their best to explain the disease to me. Type 1 Diabetes is an autoimmune disease where the body (for many reasons still unknown) suddenly recognizes its own cells as foreign and destroys them. In the case of Diabetes, it is the cells inside of the pancreas that are attacked. The pancreas is an organ located behind the stomach and is responsible for regulating the sugar in the blood. Whenever something is eaten, the body converts that food into glucose (sugar) and then uses the glucose as energy for the muscles. When too much glucose develops in the body, the pancreas secretes a hormone called insulin that processes the sugar. Too much sugar in the blood can lead to terrible complications including blindness, amputation, even death. But it's a very delicate balance, like trying to ride a unicycle on a tightrope, because not enough sugar in the blood can cause shakiness, blurred vision, and loss of consciousness.

While the two diseases have the same name, type 2 Diabetes is very different. It is usually developed in adults (while type 1 almost always occurs in people under twenty) and is the more common form of the disease. The body continues to produce insulin, but because of various factors (obesity being the foremost), the body fails to use it like it should. Thankfully, type 2 Diabetes can usually be controlled, and often times prevented, with a healthy diet and exercise.

When the doctors explained to me that I had an incurable disease that I would most likely live with for the rest of my life, it took awhile for it to sink in. It took me several days and dozens of questions to finally understand what it was that I had.

Starting that February day, I would have to check my glucose levels and give myself shots of Insulin several times every day for the rest of my life, because my body no longer made enough of its own.

Before I had my first shot, he let me practice on Babie, my beloved teddy bear that I had brought from home. He filled a syringe full of water and let me inject it into Babie's arm. Piece of cake. Mom gave me my first shot. It hurt a little. Obviously, with three shots a day, 365 days a year, I had plenty of time to get used to it.

At first, it was easy, and understandable, for me to be afraid of the needles. The idea of sticking something through my own skin was frightening to me. But the reality was that if I didn't take the shots I would die. Death has always been a great motivator for people to overcome their fears. I inject the medicine myself everyday without so much as thinking about it; but to this day, unless I am the one in control of the needle, I am still scared and disgusted to see someone else administer a shot.

I was also told that I had to test the amount of sugar in my blood by poking one of my fingers and putting the blood on a little strip. After about a minute, it would give me a number. If the number was too low (below 80) it was bad and if the number was too high (above 160) it was bad. They told me that I would have to do this several times a day, everyday, for the rest of my life.

It hit me that this disease wasn't something that was just going to go away. I wasn't going to be in the hospital for a few days and then get to go home all healthy like before. The doctors didn't know how to cure me. They just knew how to keep me alive.

After the doctor left, I remember sitting on the bed, playing Tetris on the Gameboy, while Mom sat by herself and looked out the window. Sometimes I wonder what was going on inside of her head as she sat there. Every once in awhile, she would look up at the sky and I knew what that meant: She was praying.

A couple of days later, I was allowed to go home. My life as a Diabetic started February 28, 1995. I was ten years old.

# Chapter 2
# Heal Me

*11/4/1997*
*Dear Journal,*
*This February I'll have had Diabetes for three years. I don't know what God has in store, but I wish it would happen soon. I think this is harder on Mom than on me. I can take it, but I think Mom would die if she knew this would never be lifted from me. I wish Jesus were still around so that I could touch His garment and be healed. God heal me!*

I feel that I must begin by explaining that despite what some doctors try to get us to believe, every case of this disease is not the same. There is not one rulebook to living with this disease. What works for one person may be the worst thing that could possibly be done for another. With that said, I just want to explain that the way that my parents and I chose to treat my disease is by no means meant to condemn or condone anyone. We did what we believed was best, and we must have done *something* right because, by God's grace, I'm still alive.

I love to write. If I think of something or an idea comes to mind, I write it down. I typically carry a notebook whenever I go somewhere so that I can always have something to write things down in. Although I've practiced the art of public speaking, I much prefer to put my thoughts down on paper. That way, I have more time to think about the words that are being used and can make corrections to them if needed. The written word can be an extremely powerful tool if used appropriately and I feel that the thoughts and feelings that I had concerning my disease would be communicated more clearly if I wrote them down.

This entry was written three years after I had been

diagnosed with Diabetes. It had been three years. It seems like such a long time ago, and yet the more I think about it, the more familiar and close it all seems to me.

For the first few years of having this disease, I would usually cry myself to sleep at night, thinking about what my life was like before February 28, 1995.

> *I would whisper the words to God, pleading with Him to make me better.*

After I would finally get to sleep, my mind would create these wonderful dreams; dreams where I would wake up and my blood sugar would be normal all day long, and the next day and the day after that. I would dream about how I would stop taking shots and still my blood sugar would be normal. I would dream about how, after going through three or four days, I finally realize that I have been cured! Just like that! I wasn't sick anymore! There was one time where I dreamt that I even broke out into song right in the kitchen about how I didn't have Diabetes anymore.

Then I would wake up, and realize that it had only been a dream and that I was back in the reality where I still had to take my blood and check my blood sugar levels.

I wrote this entry after praying to be cured for three years. Between my tears at night, I would whisper the words to God, *pleading* with Him to make me better. I figured that if I prayed hard, long, and *good* enough, God would eventually just take my disease away.

This entry also reveals about how I viewed my current situation. I was worried about my mom. Every time that I had a bad number, every time that she saw me longing for food that I knew I couldn't eat, every time that I had to inject that insulin into my body, she would hurt. I could see it. It seemed to hurt her deeply to know that her son had something that she could do nothing about.

It truly amazes me how I reacted to this. At only thirteen years of age, I was more concerned about my mother than I was of myself. I know that as I have gotten older I have lost some of that selflessness. It's sad really, because I know that if we all would simply take notice of others and their feelings, we would in turn help to heal our own hurts.

Honestly though, I didn't give my mother enough credit. I felt that she would just crumble if the hope for a cure were impossible. I thought that if she really knew that this disease could not be taken away from me that she would break. At thirteen years old, I hadn't yet begun to realize the incredible and enduring strength that my mother possessed.

I love my mom. She's the kind of person that whenever she is happy and in a good mood, I'm happy. When she laughs, it makes me feel good, especially when I'm the one that makes her do it. When she's sad, it really bothers me. I would try to tell a joke or make a face to make to make her forget about the thing that was making her sad. But then, something finally made her sad that I couldn't make her forget about it. It was my diabetes. It was hurting her and that was hurting me and I wasn't able to tell her that I was only joking and take that pain away.

Sometimes I wonder what my life would have been like if I had gotten this disease during Jesus' lifetime. I've read all of the passages about how the masses would come to Christ and all they would have to do was simply touch the edge of His garment. If they had enough faith, they would be cured of whatever ailed them. I used to wish so badly that I could just meet Jesus for a minute so that I could touch Him and my Diabetes would be lifted. One minute. That was all that I wanted. I just wanted to touch Him.

I ended this first entry by entreating (more like *demanding*) that God heal me of my disease. For the longest time, I viewed my diabetes as a curse, a demon that is living inside of me. I came to loathe everything about it.

It took me a while (a little too long actually) to finally come to realize something that I didn't understand when I wrote this entry. God had allowed me to experience this trial for a reason. Not as a punishment, but as something that would help me to learn some lessons. I had asked Him to cure me, but sometimes God doesn't always answer our prayers with a "yes." Sometimes He says, "no." And sometimes, He says, "wait."

# Chapter 3
# Heal Them

*11/6/1997*
*Dear Journal,*
*A few days ago, I found that Derrick had to have surgery on his ankles, because his anklebones are dying. Well, he's in casts now. We visited him two days ago and we loaned him our Sega, because he's going to be bed ridden for a while. Last time I wrote that I wanted so much to be cured of my Diabetes, but now I'd rather Derrick were able to walk than for me to be cured. Because I know I can live with it, but it would be hard for Derrick.*
*I've been praying really hard that Derrick would get better.*

In the summer of 1997 our family had moved from Bend, Oregon to Greenwood, Indiana after my dad accepted a full-time preaching position.

For the first year of living there, I really wasn't a happy camper. I still missed all of my friends that I had left back in Oregon and I was sure that I wasn't going to meet any new friends in that strange place.

In the winter of '97, we found out that Derrick, a kid from our church, was having some serious problems with his ankle bones and had to have surgery. Afterwards, he had to use crutches for a long time while his legs healed. Even after the surgery, they weren't really sure if he would be able to use his legs like he had been able to before.

I went home and really prayed about it. It was the first time that I had stopped thinking about the disease that I had been stricken with and took some time to pray about somebody else and their trouble. It made me feel good and yet, it also made me very sad, because in my mind, I figured that God only had time enough to heal a few people at a time. I told Him that if He would take the time out of His obviously busy schedule to heal Derrick, then I would quit asking Him to heal me of my disease until I knew that Derrick had been taken care of.

*11/7/1997*
*Dear Journal,*
*What I wouldn't give to have just a peek at God's overall plan. All I can do is hold on and wait. If Satan thinks my Diabetes is going to tear me down, I'll only be that much stronger. Almost three years with an incurable affliction kind of makes you forget what it was like before it came. I keep telling myself to pray for others, before I pray for myself. As long as they pull through, I don't care who it happens to. I just wish I didn't have this to distract me, when a lot of prayer needs praying. Lord! Heal them first!*

I am blown away every time I read this entry. I was openly defiant to Satan, telling myself that the harder he tried to bring me down with my Diabetes, the harder I would fight back. I was convinced that his plan would backfire and I was determined to stand my ground. I was a mere thirteen years old, but I am amazed at the zeal and the courage that I possessed at the moment that I penned these words. Even now as I enter adulthood, I can only hope that I still possess the same amazing traits that I did back then.

I've always wondered whether it would been better to have simply developed Diabetes as an infant or developed it later in life, as I had, so that I could at least enjoy a little while without the disease. If I had gotten it as an infant, I wouldn't miss anything, because I never would have experienced it in the first place. I wouldn't be saddened by all of the things that I could no longer eat or do, because I was never able to do those things to begin with. As it is, I was ten years old and fully capable to look back on my life and wish that things were back to the way that they used to be. Although I don't know which I would rather have, I do know that God allowed me to develop it at the very moment that He did, because He knew that I would be able to handle it.

It's amazing to think that because God allowed me to develop Diabetes I understood that I had an obligation to pray for others. The trouble was that now that I knew that there were so many people that needed my prayers, the same disease that had initially inspired my mission, kept distracting me and getting in the way of what I really felt that I should do. How many people have you heard say, "hold my calls, I'm going to go pray," or "please

*...having my disease for so long made it hard for me to remember what my life was like before...*

don't bother me for awhile, I've got some serious praying to do?" Many of us feel that sometimes prayer interrupts us from doing other big, important things, when all of those things that we consider so big and important are actually interrupting us from praying. Prayer (especially when we pray for others) is one of the best ways that we can use our time.

In this entry I speak of three years as being an enormous amount of time. It seems so short now. I spent the first three years waiting for the day that I would wake up and not have Diabetes anymore. It was like waiting for a special holiday that kept getting postponed. To hope and wait for something that was visible and yet never quite attainable sometimes caused me to become disappointed and frustrated.

When I say that having my disease for so long made it hard for me to remember what my life was like before, I've got to laugh at myself. Three years with Diabetes is nothing. There are many brave and courageous people that have suffered through forty years of this disease. It is true though, that after only three years, the first ten years of my life seemed blurry. It's hard for me to look past my current situation and remember how I used to be such a different person.

I can remember all the details of the day we found out that something was wrong. I can remember that I had spilled something on my T-shirt on the way to one of my brother's basketball games and how mom had rushed to the store to buy me a clean one. I can remember so many things about that day and the ones to follow, but the day before is a complete blank. The weeks leading up to it have become lost. When I talk with my siblings about the houses that we used to live in and the people that we used to know, there are times where all I can do is laugh with them and pretend to know what they're talking about, because those years before I was diagnosed seem so very far away from me.

To lose memories of when life was easier would be considered by some to be a terrible loss, but I don't see it like that. In the first few weeks after I was diagnosed, I was haunted by the previous weeks thinking, *last week I could have eaten that* or *I didn't have to worry about medicine a few days ago.* It made me angry to think of how things used to be because I knew that I was unable to go back and live in those times. When I would sleep, I would dream about how my life used to be and I would wake up angry and sad to find myself still living in my present circumstance.

> *It wasn't fair to me to keep looking back and wishing for something I couldn't have anymore.*

It wasn't fair to me to keep looking back and wishing for something I couldn't have anymore. In a way, my inability to recall some of my earliest memories was a way for me to stop living in the past and look forward to the things to come. I couldn't change the events that occurred on that day in February, but I could change the direction that my life took from that point.

Too many people hang on to the past in the hopes of somehow reliving those moments. The problem with dwelling on those things for too long is that what is happening right now passes them by with surprising speed.

What was going on at the moment of this entry was what was important. I had a friend that needed prayers far more than I did. The only complaint that I had against my disease at that point was that it was a distraction to me that kept me from doing what I knew that I needed to be doing. I needed to pray for Derrick because it was more important to me to see him walk than it was for me to not have to take my shots anymore.

*12/10/1997*
*Dear Journal,*

*A few days ago, I just lost it and started crying in Mom's lap. I haven't been doing well and I just had another really high number and that was it! Mom and I both cried and I tried to comfort her as she comforted me. She said she was sorry, but I told her not to be. This is way too hard on Mom and Dad.*

A couple of days passed since I had prayed for Derrick and I wasn't really doing very well. I tested my blood sugar and it was too high, which always made me feel like I wasn't doing a good enough job taking care of myself (which was obviously not true).

I told Mom that three and a half years was too long. When I first got Diabetes, the doctors told me that this was going to be something that I was going to have for a long time. In the mind of a then almost thirteen-year-old kid, three and a half years was an eternity. I understood that God hadn't allowed me to have this disease to punish me for anything. He allowed me to have Diabetes so that I could learn some things that I otherwise would never have been able to learn. At that point, it had allowed me to put more of my trust in God and it was actually the driving force that caused me to become a Christian. Wasn't that enough? Hadn't I learned enough so that God could finally take it away from me? But I didn't ask Him for that anymore.

I had condemned myself, but in a way I was glad. Mom had told me, "I remember when you said that you were praying for Derrick and that God would heal him and his legs before he healed you of your Diabetes. Maybe that's what God is doing, healing him before you."

It was one of those things that I had remembered doing, but didn't think anyone else had really taken notice.

When it finally dawned on me that God might very well be doing exactly what I had asked him to do, I cried. Mom held me in her arms and just let me cry. There were times that I thought I wasn't being strong enough, but what she told me that day would stay with me forever,

"You're such a little soldier, you know that?"

I didn't. I viewed myself as others typically did: a skinny, short, diabetic kid that hated looking at himself in the mirror because of the pale, sick looking figure that stared back. A soldier? Even with the wonderful imagination and creative mind that I had grown a reputation for, I never envisioned myself as such a hero.

I didn't, but she did. My mother saw me as a brave warrior who, after fighting his share of battles that most young boys his age never even face, remained steadfast and proud.

From that moment on, it no longer mattered what others thought or suggested about me. It made no difference that I was shorter, slower or weaker than anyone else.

It wasn't the fact that she told me that I was a soldier that made me feel better. She wasn't merely trying to comfort me by saying that. She was speaking from her heart as she told me something about myself that she admired. And I wasn't just anybody's soldier either. I was hers.

The tears eventually dried up, but we continued to embrace. While I was in her arms, I didn't care about anything. I didn't care about my number. I didn't care about my insulin. I didn't care about what I was going to eat for my afternoon snack. I only knew that right then my mother had given me the greatest compliment that I have ever received in my entire life.

We finally let go of each other and sat there for a while on the couch. Finally, Mom suggested that I take my blood sugar again so we could see how much insulin I would have to take. I tested it and when the number finally showed up on my little meter, we both smiled. It had dropped drastically from where it had been, back down to the normal range within only about a half an hour, without me having to take a drop of insulin. I knew then that even though I told Him that He didn't have to, God was there watching out for me.

In time, Derrick's legs healed and he was walking like nothing had happened. He was walking and I was still diabetic, and you know what? It felt good. It was an extremely fulfilling feeling. It helped to remind me that God was still there. That He answered prayers and that He still allowed His power to be seen.

I had thought that after three years, I had learned all that needed to be learned from having my disease. I was wrong. I learned that living in the past can destroy your future and selflessness was far more fulfilling than only thinking of yourself.

# Chapter 4
# My Prayer

*12/3/1997*
*Dear Lord,*

*I'm praying. I'm pleading. Just as Your Son did on the mountain before His death. Now I'm praying for a different reason. I'm losing in my battle for health. I feel I can't be a strong soldier any longer.*

*As a knight strives to free a fair maiden, I'm trying so very hard to comfort my mom and dad. I've been nicked by all of this; they've been fatally wounded.*

*I try hard to stay on my feet, while my parents carry all of our weight. I'm afraid the only stop to this unceasing fight is for me to give up. But I can hear Mom's words, "I would take it from you if I could." I'm starting to feel like a fly in a web; trapped. I need Your light in this dark cave. I need Your help.*

*Amen.*

Sometimes, as I would write in my journal, it would seem that I was doing more than writing words on a page. I was talking to someone. Often times, I would imagine that it was God that I was writing to, like writing a letter to a friend. These entries would be more than just getting my thoughts written down on a page, they would become my written prayers.

Eventually, I came to understand that God was, and always will be, there for me. He created the world in six days just by speaking, and yet He still had enough time for a little boy with Diabetes.

I'm not exactly sure what instance drove me to write this, but I know that it was a concern that continued to bother me time and time again.

Even though I was the one taking the shots, Mom and Dad were the ones that had to watch helplessly as I did it. Even though I was the one who couldn't eat the things that I really wanted to eat, Mom and Dad had to be the ones to tell me that I couldn't eat them.

I could see it on their faces. Sure, I was hurting, but they were hurting as well. At times, it seemed that their hurt surpassed my own. I hate to see my parents sad. When my parents are sad, it makes me feel miserable. During this period of my life, I was distraught because I thought that part of the reason for their sorrow was because of me.

They were the ones that had to put on a happy face for me when I knew that inside it was hurting them to see me dealing with something that they could do nothing about.

> *I was asking God to heal my parents before He healed me.*

I was asking God to heal my parents before He healed me. It's funny that in a little less than a year, I could go from begging and pleading with God to heal me, take care of me, think about me, to telling God that the only thing that I was really concerned about right then was my parents. This was one of the lessons that my disease allowed me to learn: Other people, especially my parents, are more important than myself.

The only options that I could see at that moment were to continue to watch my parents hurt by doing nothing, or to simply give into the sorrow. As I thought about it though, I came to realize that there was one more option. It came to me because of something that my mother said to me,

"I would take this disease from you if I could."

She would fight for me if it were within her power. She would sacrifice her own comfort and well being if it meant that I would not longer have to suffer. The other option that I had was to continue fighting. I could stand firm and work hard. I could choose not to let my disease get me down, because in doing so I would help encourage and strengthen my parent's resolve. They wouldn't have to be sad.

It wasn't simply a matter of working hard and doing the

things that I had to do without complaint, I had to do all of that and at the same time look at and focus on the good things that my life had to offer and be happy because of those things, instead of being sad because of this one thing.

These options apply to almost any situation in life. We can either choose to do nothing and continue to ignore the problem without confronting or resolving it; we can throw up our hands and completely give up on the problem, or we can face up to the issue and give our all in trying to improve our circumstances.

At the moment of the writing, I hadn't figured all of this out yet. I hadn't quite realized that the best way to encourage my parents was to overcome my own worry and my own sadness.

It's not to say that I never tried the first two options. I would get mad and frustrated, but I wouldn't do anything about it. I would want things to be different, but I was never willing to change anything. I was, and have always been, a creature of habit, hating the idea of change, even when I know that things will be better over the long run. I was content in my anger, because it didn't require me to do anything.

Then there were times where I would completely lose all hope. I would throw up my hands and say, "I give up." I would grow tired of trying; tired of the pain and the immense effort that I took for me to simply keep myself alive and healthy. I would shut myself away. I would rationalize that if I were unable to be cured, to claim complete victory over my disease, I would throw down my sword and refuse to fight. The only thing worse than a knight that dies in battle, is a retired knight that dies of old age.

From meeting and talking with other Diabetics, I have found most of them are trying some form of these two supposed solutions. There are those that get angry at our culture for supplying us with such unhealthy food and blame them for the development of their disease. They blame pharmaceutical companies for not trying hard enough to create a preventative treatment to keep children from getting Diabetes in the first place. Worst of all, they became filled with hate towards our God because they believe that any God that would allow His creation to suffer like we suffer must be a terrible Being indeed. They are angry with everyone and feed on their own mistrust. They complain about the horrible life that they must live, and yet are unwilling to do anything about it.

Then there are those that have completely lost all faith and hope in anything. It hurts me on the inside to see people like this. They talk about all of the pain that they must suffer and how tired they are of pressing on. They have lived with this disease for thirty, forty, fifty years and now, after trying so hard for so long, they've had enough. They resign themselves to believing that a cure will never be found and we should all just content ourselves to dying a horrible death after having a life filled with pain and disappointments. They give up. Their hope is long gone; they have faith in nothing.

I'm not saying that all Diabetics live in a state of hopelessness, but I am always surprised at just how many let this disease take all of the joy out of their lives. They create for themselves a world where their happiness is based on something that is beyond their control. Not to say that tight control over this disease is unimportant, but it wasn't because of anything that any of us did that caused us to develop this. We should not allow any kind of uncontrollable circumstances determine whether we are happy or not.

Finally, there is a type of Diabetic that I have come to recognize and they are the ones that I hope to pattern myself after. They are the ones with hope. They are the ones with faith. Whether it is faith in their doctor, faith in their own abilities or a true faith in God, they believe in something. Faith means believing in something not because we experience it with all of our senses, but because we can look back on our own experiences, know that something is going to happen, and have absolute assurance in it. I have faith that this disease will be lifted from me. Maybe not in this life, but I know that eventually I will no longer have to worry about what I eat or how much medicine I have to take. Even though I may not see the results of my faith while I'm still alive, I know that my existence will be better served and more worthwhile if I believe and look forward to that time when this disease no longer has a hold on me.

# Chapter 5
# Lifting Me Up

*12/7/1997*
*Dear Journal,*

*...Well, I just dropped and broke my R insulin. There wasn't much in it, but I still feel bad.*

*12/13/1997*
*Dear Journal,*

*"Good" news! My numbers stink and I've lost weight. The only good thing I can think of for this situation is it would take a lot more of me to reach an elevator weight limit.*

The first house that we lived in when we moved to Indiana was an old farmhouse that sat on a couple of acres. On one side of our house there was a field that usually had either corn or soy beans most of the year and the other three sides served as cow pasture. Not exactly the most pleasant of views (or smells) but it worked in keeping nosy neighbors away.

The house itself was wonderful - two stories, with plenty of bedrooms and elbowroom for our entire family. The only drawback to this home was the fact that we only had one bathroom between the eight of us (patience was a lesson well learned) and almost the entire downstairs had nothing but tile flooring. Hard, cold, tile flooring. This meant that if we ever dropped anything, we hoped to suddenly have super human reflexes, or pray that the thing that we just dropped wasn't made of glass – like my insulin vials.

I had just finished taking my first shot of the day and I was carrying my two insulin vials back to the refrigerator when my R slipped through my fingers, fell to the floor and shattered. That was enough to make me slightly upset for the rest of the morning, knowing that I had wasted some expensive medicine.

A week later, I wrote the second entry right after testing my blood and finding that it was too high and then checking my weight and finding that it was too low.

Since I can remember, I've always been skinny – even before I was diagnosed. When I got Diabetes, and my diet became more restrictive, it became hard for me to gain weight and even harder for me to keep it on.

> *.I really think that without a sense of humor, my life as a Diabetic would be miserable.*

This was the end of 1997, I was just about to turn 13 years old and I probably weighed no more than 75 pounds. Coupled with the fact that my numbers continued to be too high, I wasn't very happy.

I have always been told that the best way of dealing with something, is to look at a bad situation and try to find something good about it. Even it it's only one little thing, as long as I could find one good something about what was going on right then, I knew that eventually it was going to be all right.

This time I was stumped. What could I possibly find good about the fact that my health wasn't what it should be?

I *know* that the Lord has a sense of humor. He has to after creating something as funny as the human race. I thank Him all the time for giving me a sense of humor, too. The good thing that I found for this situation was the fact that it would take more of me to reach the weight limit in an elevator.

I didn't realize it then, but my sense of humor – my ability to laugh and also make other people laugh – is probably one of the things that have allowed me to keep going. When I tell a joke or do my John Wayne impression and make somebody laugh, the fact that the joke was told by a Diabetic isn't going to make any difference. I have chosen not only to laugh in spite of my disease, but just as with this instance, I have chosen to laugh because of my disease. I can't tell you how many "drug" jokes I've made with my friends as I prepare to inject my insulin. I really think that without a sense of humor, my life as a Diabetic would be miserable.

Even so, I was still feeling down about the way things were going. Once again, I forgot that God was there with me. He was there when my high number appeared on my glucose monitor, he was there when I stepped onto the bathroom scale, and He had something special waiting for me.

*12/23/1997*
*Dear Journal,*

*...I had another good number this morning! I've been having good numbers in the mornings for a few days! I don't know how we do it; I just want it to continue!*

Only a week after I was complaining about my high numbers, I wrote about how my morning numbers had been doing great! Some people may not think that this was any big deal, but since I was first diagnosed, I always had trouble keeping my numbers from mysteriously rising during the night. I may go to sleep with a perfectly normal number and yet wake up to find that it had jumped while I was asleep. Some refer to this as the Dawn Phenomenon.

It seems to me that God looked down on me and realized that I needed a little bit of something to cheer me up. It wasn't anything supernatural, but it was enough to get my spirits back up and get me out of the rut of self-pity that I had gotten myself into.

This is something that I find myself doing from time to time. When bad things happen to me in quick succession, I don't have time enough to step back, calm my nerves, and muster up some strength to get through it. Instead, I keep taking the hits and covering the pain, until I simply can't anymore. I often times become so overwhelmed with things that have happened months before, and because I haven't taken the time to deal with them, I still carry their weight.

When hard times come because of my disease (or anything else for that matter) I need to take a deep breath and evaluate how I can best deal with the situation, instead of letting it eat away at me.

# Chapter 6
# I'll Be Like Job

*11/2/1998*
*Dear Journal,*

*God works in mysterious ways all right. Mom, Dad and I are the only people I know who are trying to get rid of my Diabetes, while everyone one else just "lives with it." And for everything we've done for my body, I seem to be worse than I was when I was first in the hospital. But, I know God has a plan and He's watching out for me. I'll be like Job. Even if I have an incurable affliction overtake my body, it will only make me pray more and lean on God more than ever. Diabetes was the reason I was baptized. God's plan had brought forth some fruit already!*

I believe that the first part of this entry deserves some explanation. The thing that I most remember about the doctors and nurses while I was in the hospital was how they kept telling me what I had and how I could best "deal with it." They never really offered me any solutions to my problem. My problem was Diabetes, but all they could do was tell me the details about what my problem was and how best to keep it from killing me. They never told me how to get rid of it or even how to hope to try.

"This is your life now," they told me. "You're going to have to change some things about how you eat and take care of yourself. You have Diabetes now, and there is no known cure for that. This is your life, deal with it."

It was like they just plopped a heap of stinking manure in my lap and told me that this was how things were going to be, that I had to "deal with it," and that I shouldn't even bother trying to figure out how to get this dung off of me. I should merely accept that I was now living with something that couldn't be taken away.

Let's just say that I could never see any of them making a career out of motivational speaking.

It had been almost four years. It was true, I was living with an incurable disease, but neither my parents nor I were ever willing to simply "deal with it" and content ourselves with treating the symptoms and not try to cure the disease.

I'm not sure when we first went, but when my family and I were still living in Bend, Oregon, my mom took me to a naturopathic physician named Dr. Mark Cooper. He had a reasonably good-sized office in town where he practiced herbal medicine and acupuncture.

There were a lot of different things that I liked about Dr. Cooper, but the one thing that I will always love him for was that he was the first person that I could remember since being diagnosed that tried to offer me some hope.

After living a few years with Diabetes, hope was now becoming more than just a word to me. It was something that I longed for; something that I needed to survive.

My parents and I used to spend hours talking with Dr. Cooper in his office about how I was doing, new herbs that I might be able to try, just all sorts of things. Sometimes we wouldn't talk about my disease at all; we would just talk about everyday things. I loved talking to him, because he always smiled when he looked at me. I loved the fact that to him I was more than just another patient that came into his office with a bunch of problems – I was somebody. He treated me like somebody important. The things that mattered to me and to my parents mattered to him. At this time, the thing that mattered most to us was finding a cure to my Diabetes and so he did what he could to help and encourage us towards that end.

I believe that some of the things that he told me during the time that I spent with him helped me more than any herbal remedy ever did.

He told me that a lot of times our own well being is determined by the attitude that we have about life. If we're down and depressed all of the time and we think that the world is just a horrible place - that everything bad is happening to us because we're just a lowly nobody - we're probably not going to be as healthy as the person who has a positive outlook on life. My attitude will, in part, help determine how I feel.

The other thing that he did that I greatly appreciated was that instead of just trying to get me to accept that I was doomed to a life of endless tests and shots, he told me that he sincerely believed that a cure for Diabetes would come within my lifetime. He told a twelve-year-old boy that one day he might live to see the end of this disease. He probably doesn't even realize it, but that has stayed with me to this day. The best thing about it was that he wasn't simply telling me that to make me feel better, he really believed it and that's what made him so wonderful.

*He wasn't simply telling me that to make me feel better, he really believed it.*

Doctor Cooper had me try a lot of different things – pills, tinctures, acupuncture, most of which helped me feel healthier and maintain a good complexion and steady weight. Before I met Doctor Cooper, I was really looking very sickly. I was extremely pale and thin and I had these huge circles underneath my eyes. Nowadays I hate to look at pictures of myself during that time because I looked like death itself.

After only a few months of going to Doctor Cooper, I was looking and feeling good. I felt good inside because not only was he helping me to improve my health, he had succeeded in improving my spirits. He gave me hope, and that was something that I had a very short supply of up until that point.

Despite all of the wonderful things that he did for me, something had briefly happened to me doing this time that caused my numbers to skyrocket and my mom and I were having a difficult time keeping them under control. Because of that, I was getting discouraged.

Thankfully, my belief and faith in God (the One Who created my body) was strong enough that I still realized that He was in control and that He was obviously preparing me for something good to come out of the bad that I was currently experiencing. As time went on that became a good motivation for me. When things got bad, I just told myself that something good must be coming.

The bad things were there so that I would be able to recognize the good when it arrived.

It didn't take me very long to understand that good things had already come because of it, but it would take a little while for me to fully realize how important this good would be for me.

For the time being, I just decided to grit my teeth and bear it as best as I could. I would imitate Job from the Bible. The man lost his entire family (except sadly for his nagging unbelieving wife), his property, his livestock, his physical health, his friends, and the list goes on. All I had to worry about was a physical disease; I didn't have to scrape the sores of my leprosy with broken pottery like Job did. Compared to him, my life was a cakewalk. I wasn't going through half of what that man must have had to, so I wasn't about to let this little thing lick me.

*7/7/2002*
*Dear Journal,*

*One day. Just one day. If someone had to live a 24-hour period inside of my mind, it would break them like it has almost broken me.*

*My brain does not function like a regular person's would. I have to create logic while sifting through the poisoned thoughts and ideas that come rushing through my head. This poison is like a black cloud that slowly spreads. Sure, they told me that It would affect my muscles; the blood would rush to my fingertips. I could handle that. Sure, no problem. But did they ever think about how it might affect my mind?*

*Will I get picked on today?*

*What do I say when someone moans and tells me that it must really stink to be me?*

*How do I react when someone holds a sugar-filled something up to my face, licks their lips and says. "MMM! This is so good?"*

*Who will I yell at today while under the influence of high blood sugar?*

*How will I react when someone ignorantly fills my diet Coke up with regular? Will I just forget it and throw the drink away or will*

*I get into their face and let them know that they had filled my drink up with a deadly poison? They could have killed me!*

*What do I tell my parents when I argue with them for no reason other than the fact that while my number is soaring anything that they say to me will set me off?*

*Most people don't have to think about whether they will wake up in the morning. Nobody should have to think about that. Nobody should have to suffer like that. Nobody should have to always wish for Heaven to come during the night so that they don't have to wake up in the morning and face another day. Nobody should, but I do.*

*I will still praise the Lord in this. I will be like Job.*

This entry was written years after I had first compared myself to Job, but the idea still remained. Job was such a cool dude. Even though he had a bunch of people around him, including his wife, telling him how awful he must have been to have ticked God off so bad, he was still able to look ahead and know that God had a purpose for him. He never faltered; he never stopped believing in God, even though it seemed to some that God had abandoned him.

A lot of things were going on in my head when I was writing this. At that time I was having a hard time dealing with the fact that some people were telling me how they thought I should be reacting to my disease. They were telling me that I really shouldn't be making such a big deal about the little things that came along with having Diabetes – the name calling, the ridicule, the torment. "What's the big deal?" they would ask me.

I guess that this entry was my way of trying to disprove them. It was me telling myself why I did things, justifying my actions by exploring my thought process. True, I do not think that I can use the excuse of having Diabetes every time that I do something stupid; that wouldn't be fair. But I do believe that some people don't consider what a Diabetic has to think about every day of their lives; Things that a person without it would never have to give a second thought to.

I know of someone who used to find it amusing to make fun of me and my disease for the same reason that many people make fun of others: he didn't understand it. It was really starting to get to me how people would say and do things and never think about how it might affect the feelings of someone like me, someone "different." Thankfully, this same person now understands and appreciates what Diabetics have to go through and acknowledges the courage that it takes to do it and still be happy.

It's true, we Diabetics have to deal with things that other people don't, but that doesn't make us better than anybody. Everybody has their own unique struggles that they have to deal with. That's life. We should just remember that the way we deal with those struggles is what defines our character.

*The next time that you feel you're being tested, just remember Job.*

I don't want others looking down on me because of my disease and I don't look down on others who may not know how to deal with something like this. It doesn't make me any better or worse than the next guy.

Job didn't boast about his determination. He didn't rub into his friend's faces the fact that he was simply being tested instead of punished like they tried to convince him. He remained humble about it and did only what was expected of him by God.

The next time that you feel you're being tested, just remember Job and realize that if he could get through the death of all of his children, the destruction of his property and the loss of his entire livelihood and yet remain true and faithful to God, then whatever you're going through should seem like a walk in the park.

# Chapter 7
# Death Came For Me

*1/2/2002*
*The War Inside Me*

It is something that haunts and torments me almost every waking hour, and if I allow it to consume me, I am certain that it will destroy me.

I have to write quickly before its effects begin to wear off. February 2002 will mark seven long years that I've had to live with a demon inside me. Four years ago it almost killed me, and I'll never be the same carefree, adventurous artist that I used to be.

My vision wavers even as I write this. That's something new, but I know what to attribute it to. The same power that makes my hands shake and my temper flare. The same thing that magnifies my pain but dulls my other senses.

It's my Diabetes. My thorn in the flesh.

I'm more aware of it now, as I am about many other things. Its presence seems to hover over my soul and plague me from the inside. It's always there, keeping me from using the common sense that I know I need, but just can't seem to get at.

In a matter of minutes comes the feeling of blood rushing to my head, my toes and the tips of my fingers. Anxiousness, impatience and intolerance will just as quickly rush over me. The faults and disappointments of myself and others will immediately become evident. My mouth will move faster than my brain and the thought of what effect my words will have on others will only become clear after the thing has been spoken. Too much anger spoken too often.

It's as if I've become intoxicated. No, it must be worse, because I can feel it coming and I still have a sense of control. I still have control and that's what drives me out of my mind. It's not just the disease that often makes me feel and act and think the way I do. At least not all by myself. It's me! It would be easy for me to simply say, "my number is high and that is why..." I chewed your head off or secluded myself from the group or grabbed you and pushed you backwards up over the couch.

These are my *thoughts* and my *feelings simply magnified* by my unseen enemy.

But now I take a breath and pause as the poison hand of this sickening tormentor releases its death grip upon my mind and heart.

I have today because my ever-present and all-knowing Creator chose to spare my life from the chains of death that this evil had on me those many years ago. Many, but not quite so many.

It is still pressed to the front of my memory. I still remember the words that I spoke as I was taken to the hospital in the arms of my older brother. I asked what Heaven would be like. I told him that I was ready. I was ready. Ready to meet my Creator. But it wasn't God's will that my end should come just then.

I often ask the reason why I was spared. Why I was given another chance. Why? Why me? Obviously it was not from anything that I had done to deserve the mercy of my God. The reason was simply this.

He had plans for me.

So here I am complaining about the effects and feelings that I must endure, when I should be thankful that I'm even able to feel anything at all. God could have taken me, but He didn't.

The battle rages ever on, but this young warrior is not so easily broken. I simply have to defeat myself first.


Diabetes has been known to affect your eyes. It's one of the more common problems associated with this disease. When my number would soar, my vision would suddenly blur. It would only be like that for a split second, but it would be enough for me to know that something wasn't right. As I wrote this entry, I was having trouble focusing on the words, so I just wrote as fast as I could without really concentrating on what I was writing.

Often times, when I knew that my blood sugar was too

high, I would write in my journal as I waited for my insulin to kick in. The effects of my high blood sugars were becoming more apparent and I would try and write down how I was feeling at the very moment, knowing that in a little less than fifteen minutes, my sugar would be normal again and I would hardly remember why exactly I had been feeling so angry, so wound up, so *insane* only moments before.

It was something that I struggled with for a long time. Most people would tell me that I'm a pretty mild mannered sort of guy. I try to use common sense and I don't really like getting into arguments. Since developing Diabetes, I had to get used to a whole new side of my personality. The trouble was that for a while I refused to acknowledge that it really was me doing these things.

From the very beginning, my blood sugar would affect my attitude. The first few years, if my blood sugar was too high, it would cause me to get very depressed. I thought that my number was high because I wasn't taking good enough care of myself. It was high because I ate that extra pancake or didn't take enough insulin or I hadn't exercised like I should have. It was high and it was all my fault.

Before long though, my family was able to recognize another change in me due to my blood. I would get angry very easily. I would snap at my siblings for no real reason at all. Other things started happening to me as well. Not only would my temper be affected, but I would also experience heightened senses. Sounds that I heard everyday would suddenly become louder and more irritating. Along with this came a heightened sense of pain. A simple way that I could tell if my blood was too high was if I stubbed my toe. Sometimes just bumping into a desk or tripping over something would hurt so much I was hardly able to breathe!

Anger is not an uncommon symptom of high blood sugar. Each Diabetic reacts to too much sugar in their own different way and anger was usually mine. I've joked about creating a comic book character much like the Hulk, except it wasn't some science experiment gone wrong that would cause me to go ballistic, it was my lack of insulin.

When I refer to how I might push someone backwards over the couch, I speak of an incident that happened when I was about seventeen. There was a teen get-together at our house one Sunday evening. Our family often invited the teens from our church to come over to our house to play games and have Bible studies. There was one guy who (supposedly "out of fun") decided to put me into one of those strange arm holds and knock me down. He was older and bigger so, obviously, I hit the floor square on my back. He was laughing. I wasn't. Without even thinking, I sprung on him, pushed him back up and over our couch and just held him there. I then said, very softly,

"Don't do that again."

He was shocked. I was too. Apparently, so were several other people in the room. It was typical for me to be on the receiving end of silly jokes and pranks, but it was completely out of my character to ever retaliate in a physical way. I knew immediately that my number was out of whack. The adrenaline rush and strength came with its side effects: an extremely short fuse.

*From the very beginning, my blood sugar would affect my attitude.*

We eventually laughed it off and went on with the evening, but I still remember that evening thinking, *whoa, did I really do that?* It was frightening because my lack of insulin would suddenly, and often times without any warning whatsoever, change my personality into someone that I didn't like. I suppose that's really why I began referring to my Diabetes as "the demon inside of me." Whenever my numbers would get high, it was like someone other than me would make himself known through my anger.

I was really having a hard time when I wrote this entry, because it seemed that I wasn't able to go a day without blowing my top at someone or getting overly annoyed by some little thing.

The strangest thing of all was when I would get into an argument or discussion during these times. In my head, I would be able to make the most complete perfect logic that I figured any human being could possibly come up with, but when it finally got around to saying it and expressing it to others, it didn't make sense at all. It's like my thoughts would get scrambled and I wouldn't be able to keep track of where they were all going. I would continue to press my point of view until I was completely exasperated and left or my number returned to normal. I would be truly convinced that my point of view was the correct one and I would refuse to let it go, even though everyone could see that I was mistaken.

This was a big deal for me. It was what was driving me crazy, because I would try to make excuses for myself and just say that it was my blood sugar that was making me act that way. Eventually, I had to come to realize that my excuse wasn't going to work forever. I had to start taking responsibility for my own actions. It was *my* Diabetes that was causing me to do what I was doing, so it was up to me to make sure that I didn't allow my attitude to be affected. Obviously, this took me quite some time to figure out and I still struggle with it. I just had to finally realize that it wasn't *just* my disease that was making me do these things, it was me as well. "Defeating myself" is something that I must constantly remind myself to do, but at least I don't have to feel alone. We all have to "defeat ourselves." Our human instinct is often dangerously far from what we actually should to do. If we all automatically knew how to do the right thing, we would no longer need the wisdom and guidance that we all search for. Often times, we must overcome and best our own human desires to make the right decision.

*"God could have taken me, but He didn't."* At the age of ten I was forced to face the fact that I now had something that could very well claim my life. When I tell people that I have Diabetes, a lot of them tell me how sorry they feel for me.

"Man, that must be rough."

"That must really stink."

At first, that's what I wanted people to say. Yeah, it *is* rough! It *does* stink! Life sure would be a lot better if I didn't have this disease! What I was really saying was that life sure would be better if I was someone else; someone other than Craig.

These many years later, I have to stop myself. I have to quit looking through my self-inflicted tunnel vision. I have to look past the shots, the finger pricks, and the missed desserts and see what this disease has done to me, what this disease has done for me.

When people try to tell me that they feel sorry for me, I don't really blame them. It's common human reasoning to think that current, immediate suffering must be uncomfortable and sometimes they're right. I just smile at them. The point isn't merely that I have a disease; it is what has happened to me because I have it. Mortality isn't just for old people. I know that death will eventually come, so why should I have to worry about where I'll be going after death?

*That's* why God allowed me to have this disease. He knew that this would eventually bring me to think about death, and cause me to ask myself whether or not I was ready for it when it came.

I once told my mom that I was glad that God had allowed me to have Diabetes. Crazy, huh? I know, I know, you're probably thinking, *what? Are you out of your mind? Why in the world would you be glad to have something like this?*

Mom didn't say that. She just quietly let me express my thoughts without interruption. I told her I was glad because if I hadn't been inflicted with an incurable disease, the thought of dying would never have come up at that point in my life. I was ten years old for crying out loud! I wasn't going to die! I had at least a hundred years left to go, right? Up until that time I had always thought that preparing for death was something that big people did. Older people did that because they were getting old. They had to think about where they would go when they died. Not me. No, no. I was only ten; I still had years and years to go before I even had to worry about all of that Heaven and Hell, do-you-know-where-you're-gonna-go kind of stuff.

Less than two years after I was diagnosed I sat in church one Wednesday night, so completely preoccupied in my own thoughts that I didn't hear a single word the speaker was saying. I had already heard it a thousand times before. It would have been nice to say that the message that this man brought was the reason that I decided to follow Christ and be baptized, but it wasn't. Believe it or not, at 12 years of age, I was worried about what would happen to me when I died. I knew that I had a disease that claimed thousands of lives each year. I told my parents, "If this disease is going to kill me, I wanted to be ready for it when it does." I was baptized and saved the very next morning.

I could not have chosen a better time. Within one year of coming to Christ, I was almost called away to be with Him. Within a 24-hour period, I went from lying on the couch with a really bad side ache to lying on a hospital bed not realizing then, that I had come within two hours of death.

I had a bad reaction to some medication that I had just started taking. When that happened, my body was dangerously low on potassium, causing me to hallucinate and, in essence, temporally go out of my mind. I yelled and screamed things at my family; things that I didn't really mean or understand, but just seemed to come out of me as my mind and body shut down. I don't exactly understand all of the medical jargon for what happened, but the long and short of it is that my body was reacting to the pain without conscious direction from my brain.

I remember very little of that day. It was like I was walking around in one of those dreams where everything around me was moving very slowly, while at other times things were going so fast that I could hardly get my bearings.

It was a Saturday morning and all of us kids had gone downstairs into the living room to watch cartoons. After about an hour or so, my back started to ache. It was like someone was grabbing a muscle back there and pinching it as hard as they could. I tried changing my position on the floor. The pain remained. I drank some water, because sometimes my back would hurt when I didn't drink enough. The pain increased like nothing I had ever felt. I went into the bathroom and sat on the floor, closing my eyes and wishing that the pain would just go away.

My family realized it was more than a backache when I couldn't get up off of the bathroom floor. I was enveloped in pain. After calling Dr. Cooper, and trying various remedies without any results, my mother realized that she had to bring me in as fast as possible. She quickly wrapped me in a blanket and had my older brother, Jeremy, carry me to the van. I lay in his lap, as Mom sped to Dr. Cooper's office.

The conversation that I had with my older brother on the way to the doctor's office was one of the few memories that I have of that day. I think that there's a reason for that. Still dazed and confused, I had asked him,

"What will Heaven be like?"

I don't know if I got an answer from him or whether I have

simply forgotten it, but I remember repeating over and over, "I'm ready. I'm ready to go. I'm ready."

I was ready. I was ready to go home to my Father. My mind was almost completely shut down, but my spirit, it seems, knew exactly what was going on. My body was just about to die, but my spirit was getting ready to *finally* live.

Sometimes I think about what I might have mumbled on the way to the doctor, if I hadn't already given my life to Him. Would I have had the confidence that I had at that moment? The confidence of knowing exactly where I was going? I didn't ask Jeremy whether I would get to go to Heaven or not, I asked him what it would be like when I got there. The only thing that I thought about on the way to the doctor was the only thing that was really worth thinking about. As far as I could tell, I was going to die that day. I didn't ask where I would be going. I was sure of my destination. I just wanted to know more about it before I got there.

I remember briefly arriving at Dr. Cooper's office. I was set on the table and I remember thinking to myself as everything went to black, *I can't breathe.*

The next thing I knew, I was slowly waking up in a hospital with both of my parents sitting at the foot of the bed. I hadn't had any out of body experience. I didn't see the face of Jesus in the clouds. It was more like I had just woken up from a horrible nightmare, except that when I looked around the room and saw the white linens, heard the beeping monitors, and felt the I.V. in my arm, I knew that it had not been a nightmare. It had all been real.

Death had come for me. He had sat beside me and whispered my name, and yet for some reason, he had been called away.

*2/5/2001*

Dear Journal,

"Fear God and keep His commandments, for this is man's all." No matter what this world tries to throw at me, I must always remember that this world is just a shadow. It isn't real. Heaven is the only real thing.

I've started to notice during the past few months that my life, my actions, what I say and do...it just seems that I'm only walking around in a dream. I'm always strangely aware that this entire physical world isn't real. This world's joys are too short and the disappointments too long. I'm walking in a bubble...waiting for something that is real. I know that the thing that I long for is my Heavenly home. God is real.

I feel that God has put me on earth for a purpose. I'm a chess piece, sitting, waiting for the Master to move me where He wills.

I can no longer disappoint Him (or myself). I must strive as hard as ever to be the strong, faithful soldier that God expects of me. Sometimes it seems that the world is trying to choke me with its deathly cold hands always around my neck. But what kind of strength does that world have on me? None! The pressure may rise, the responsibility may seem like too much, but the world's hands will simply weaken their grip on me every time that I remember that I am here for a reason.

It would have been too easy for me to have gone home with God those years ago when Death got so close. But no! I'm still here and I'm not leaving until I've changed the world! I'm not even here for me anymore. God decided that I should remain alive, so the life that I have remaining will be given to God. Fair enough!

So for all of those rash thoughts, temptations, angry words or any other sins that dare defy my God, I will prove to them and every human being that lives on this earth, that Craig Dehut isn't leaving until his mission of changing the world for the better has successfully been accomplished!

I didn't fully comprehend the full extent of my ordeal those many years ago until I was talking about it with my mom one day. Sometimes I'll ask her questions about that day because for the most part, I only really remember a couple of short moments. At times, I couldn't see anything, even though my eyes were open. I could only hear what was going on around me. My lack of fluid was effecting how much blood was getting to my brain. My brain was shutting down like a malfunctioning computer.

Mom told me about how one of the doctors had said that it was a good thing that they had brought me in when they had, because I was about two hours away from death. That really kind of woke me up to what had really happened. It wasn't time for me to leave. The more I think about it, the more I question the reason why. Why had I been saved? I quickly realized why I *hadn't* been saved. Whenever I did something I knew I shouldn't, whenever I disappointed my parents, my siblings or my God, I would know that I was not saved so that I could sin. God had preserved me for something far greater.

What is my reason for being right now? Simple. I owe God more than I know I can ever repay: my life, my parents, and my hope. I know that the only thing I can do is try my utmost to make myself worthy of the gift.

2/1/2002
*Dear Journal,*

*This is the month of my "anniversary." Seven years ago this month, I was diagnosed with Diabetes. When it happened I thought that my life was over, but it's been so long since I wasn't a Diabetic that I can't really imagine myself without it. All of my memories before that time seem so far away.*

*I used to cry myself to sleep every night during the first couple of years. Crying and praying that God would heal me. I prayed that I didn't understand nor deserve the punishment that God had dealt to me. I didn't understand at first, but I finally came to realize that I wasn't be punished, I was being tested.*

*I think that a feeling of peace finally came over me after my Diabetes almost took my life. It was my third year, I think, and the odds were against me. After that day – to which I still can hardly recall – I knew that there was a reason that God had given me a second chance. I didn't want to waste it.*

*2/27/2002*
*Dear Journal,*

*Tomorrow will mark the day that my life changed forever. It can't be undone and, at present, it can't be fixed. I'm just left to keep carrying on, as I watch time tick away.*

*Seven years. It almost seems unreal. I can remember those days clearly: The trip over the mountain and the half a dozen stops that I had to make. Mom taking me to the doctor, suspecting a simple infection, but fearing something worse. It almost seems that she knew that something was going to happen. The way that she looked me with those sad eyes and held my hand as we sat in the waiting room.*

*I remember coming home so that I could grab a couple of things and then leave again. The other kids were watching Mary Poppins. None of them really understood what was going on. I didn't even fully understand. But I did understand that I was sick, and no one knew how to make it better.*

*Jeff let me take his Gameboy with me, so that I would have something to do while I was in the hospital. I played games while Mom would sit by the window and stare outside. I had become sick in my body, but Mom had become sick in her heart. Neither of us would ever fully recover.*

*Now here I am, seven years later. I've taken countless shots, I've swallowed countless pills, and I've seen countless doctors. I'm still sick in the body, but we're no longer sick in the heart.*

*Four years ago, I had a wake up call. God almost took me home. I was ready, but God had other plans. Better plans.*

*A cure seems just around the corner. Will I live to see it and be relieved of my disease? To me, it doesn't really matter now. Live or die, either way, my curse will no longer have a hold on me.*

Death came for me, but God told him to wait. Now I can only try to do everything within my power to prove that saving me had actually been worth His time.

# Chapter 8
# Look for the Good

*11/4/1998*
*Dear Journal,*

*Boy! I feel like I'm behind on everything! Or maybe I'm trying to get everything done at once. I have this flawed belief that everything in my life has to flow, to work just right. But I'm reaching for the impossible. My Diabetes made quite a few bumps in my path, but after awhile some good came out of it. So I figure I had better set straight what has to be done now, and realize what should be left for later. And if something that I don't see coming suddenly makes my life a little rocky, I'll just find some way to use it for good, and not stumble over the rocks.*

I hate to waste time. I'm the sort of guy that likes to work out in my mind what I want to get accomplished for the next day before I go to sleep at night. *Okay, I want to do this and this and this and I'm going to spend this much time on this so that I'll still have a chance to do this.* I guess it's just the way I am. Call me a perfectionist if you like, I just hate standing around and thinking, *I could be doing something much more productive right now.*

I wrote this as we were coming up on the holiday season. In other words, I was getting into that certain time of the year when things *never* go exactly like you plan them. You may have a perfect picture of what you want your day to look like, and then boom! Reality happens.

I was feeling a bit overwhelmed with it all - dealing with all of the regular troubles that I usually bring upon myself coupled together with my Diabetes - I was starting to feel the stress. After I had complained about it, I stepped back, as I usually found myself doing, and realized that life in general *never* goes the way you think it will either.

Things are going to go wrong. It happens. I personally did not plan on getting Diabetes when I was ten years old; it wasn't scheduled in my life's daily planner. It still happened though and I was forced to figure out the best way to deal with it. As is always the case with things like this, something that I expected would eventually ruin my life caused some good things to happen.

An idea that I express in this entry is something that is worth mentioning. When something bad happens, it is reasonable to expect that something good will come from it. Whether it is that you learn patience or endurance or that you help to strengthen another by your example, something good may come from it. It may not come right away (my years with Diabetes continue and I'm just now coming to realize the good), but it will eventually come.

The idea that I wanted to get across when I said that I would *"just find some way to use it for good"* was that we shouldn't expect the good to just fall into our laps. We have to be the ones to use this inconvenience and *use* it to find the good. Finding the good means that we have to step outside of our comfort zone and look for it! Often times, the good has been there all along, we just never looked far enough to see it.

One of the best things that I have realized from my getting this disease is this: I am thankful that God allowed me to have Diabetes, *instead* of allowing someone else in my family to have it.

I pause for a moment and consider that. I have it and they do not. It would be very hard to have to watch one of my siblings suffer through the things that I have had to suffer through without being able to do anything about it. It is so wonderful that my God chose to let me have it. At first I didn't want to believe it, but I now I know that He let it happen to me because He knew that I could handle it.

Diabetes was a "bump." It was an imperfection in the perfect world that I was constantly trying, and failing, to create for myself. It's an impossible goal, as I have finally begun to realize, but it has bettered me. God has allowed me to see the good in even something as horrible as Diabetes.

I tell myself that I should get in order the things that I know need to be dealt with now and leave the things that can be left alone until later.

This entry was written the same year that I decided to become a Christian. Leaving uncertain my fate after death was obviously something that I simply could not save until later. It was something that I needed to consider and act on.

Recently, I woke in the middle of the night with my blood sugar lower than it's ever been. I have never felt so panicked. I was at a friend's house, sleeping on the couch downstairs. Everyone else was upstairs. I stumbled off of the couch and found my glucose tablets, popped two of them in my mouth and frantically gulped a glass of water.

I stood in the kitchen and shook. Mostly because of the lack of sugar in my blood (uncontrolled shaking is a common symptom), but also because I realized that I had been lucky enough to wake myself with low sugar. I could have remained asleep and continued sleeping until I finally passed out. No one would have known. Even if someone had come downstairs, I would have looked like I was still just sleeping.

It was very sobering. I am thankful to God that I chose to follow Him those many years ago. "If this disease is eventually going to kill me, I want to be ready for it when it does."

I was getting my life ready for death so that, eventually, I would be able to have life with Him. Life suddenly made my road a little rocky when I was ten years old, but I have found so many ways to turn it into something wonderful. I looked for the good and found it.

# Chapter 9
# The Demon Inside of Me

*2/25/1999*
*Dear Journal,*

*Picture this: A man on death row with only a few weeks left. But in the back of his mind he has a hope of getting out, however slim the chance.*

*The past couple months have been a whirlwind of emotions, thoughts and fears. When my blood sugar levels get too high, it seems that I fall into major depression. I know this is better than lashing out at other people. Now I'm only hurting myself and no one else.*

*But it's much harder than that. It's like being intoxicated. I can't think straight, all that I can comprehend is that whatever has just happened to me is the worst thing that could have happened to me, and it's all my fault.*

*Then there are those times when my blood sugar is where it's supposed to be and it's like getting a breath of fresh air! And I hang onto the slim chance that I'll finally be set free from the prison that I've made of my own self.*

*Even though it seems rough sometimes (more times than I think it should), God still gives me my fresh air. And I wait for Heaven: God's eternal air!*

Because of my personality, I always like to envision things a certain way. I plan out in my mind what I would like to get accomplished that day and try my very best to get it done. That's not a bad thing. I think that it is very constructive if you set goals for yourself. I believe that we should never be content with the way that we are, we should always be striving to improve and better ourselves. The problem with my outlook at the time of this entry was that I would plan and set goals for myself, but I would become severely depressed when things didn't work out just the way that I wanted them to.

Take my blood sugar numbers for example. Obviously, they're supposed to be within a certain range – not too high and not too low. When they would get too high, I would blame myself for it and would become upset that my numbers hadn't turned out the way that I had planned.

As I write about this now, I have to laugh at myself. As anyone who knows this disease understands, there will be times when your blood sugar isn't going to be within the range that has been set for you. It happens. You take some insulin and get some exercise to bring it down or you eat a snack to bring it back up. You just fix it and go on with your life, without beating yourself up every time it gets a little out of whack.

Through this time in my life, I was often getting very depressed and discouraged whenever my number wasn't where I really wanted it to be. My parents and my siblings would commonly have to remind me, "Come on. It's not the end of the world. Don't let it get you so down."

I would blame myself for my number and although the level of control with this disease comes from always being aware of how you feel and making sure that you stay on top of it, it wasn't fair of me to blame and get upset with myself for the fact that I did have something that was, in a way, out of my hands.

*2/27/2002*
*Dear Journal,*


*I'm fighting against myself. If my numbers are high, I get grumpy, snappy and angry! I'll get upset at everyone for doing everything.*

*I'm writing now, because I'm doing just that right now. I'm mad at the world, for no good reason. I'm having trouble breathing, sleeping, and my temper! When I first got Diabetes, I never figured I would have to go through this, or anyone else (Mom and Dad) would have to go through this.*

*For now, I'm waiting for my insulin to start working, so I won't be so mad. And I'm still waiting for something to turn things around for me. I'm hoping, I'm praying, I'm waiting...*

> *I realized that I couldn't let my blood sugar effect me in such a negative way.*

As any diabetic knows, mood swings are a common side effect of high blood sugar. Other symptoms include excessive thirst and urination, tired limbs, etc., but as far as my experience went, I could always tell when my blood sugar was too high, because I would allow the demon inside of me to emerge.

I came to realize that blaming myself and getting upset and depressed about my disease was not only useless, it *never* improved my situation, but was instead destructive. It was destroying my sense of happiness. I firmly believe that God allowed me to have this disease. God is One who wishes for us to be happy, truly happy, even when we don't desire it for ourselves. I'm not going to let something like a disease take His joy away from me.

Instead of taking these disappointments out on myself, I started directing them towards my family, which I believe had more of a destructive effect on everyone and really just made the problem worse.

Normally, I'm a pretty even keeled kid. I usually don't get too excited or adamant about anything, so it was always very apparent to those around me that my number was too high because I would just come unglued about the littlest of things. Often times my pulse would begin to race, regular light would become blinding to me, everyday sounds would become higher pitched and annoying.

When I finally wrote down this entry, I was trying desperately to capture and express how I was feeling at the very moment, because as soon as my number would return to normal, I really wouldn't be able to comprehend why exactly I had been so upset, or why I had felt the way that I had felt.

This happened quite often. There were days that I must have been just horrible to be around. It wasn't fair to my family that they had to suffer through these times. I realized that I couldn't let my blood sugar effect me in such a negative way. Sure, it was going to get too high sometimes, but it was still up to me as to how it was going to affect my attitude.

2/11/2002
*Dear Journal,*

*The reason. What was the reason? At times it comes to me so clear, other times I'm left in a fog. What was the reason? What does it mean? Why was I chosen?*

*Why was I chosen to bear something and others are left untouched? How come the only memories that I'm left with are the ones with that shadow constantly hanging over me? Sometimes I try to recall how my life was before I was cursed, but I can't. Nothing comes to me anymore. That part of me has died, lost to the Shadow.*

*Surely there was someone more capable, more prepared, to handle this. Why was I the one?*

*A day doesn't go by when I'm not keenly aware of its presence. It's always there. It's like that feeling of having someone stalking you. You know that they're going to eventually find the right time and place and then take hold of you and never loosen their cold fingers from your neck.*

*Things go on in my mind that I don't understand; things that I can't explain. Is it really me thinking these thoughts or is it the deadly poison of my Stalker, cunningly trying to wear away at my sanity until I finally go out of my mind by attempting to evade the madness?*

*What was the reason? I don't think that the true answer is what I want to hear. There may have never been a reason! Satan could have been allowed to torment me with my own self, now under the influence of a little monster living inside of me, just for the fun of it! My God would never have done that to me. I will not curse God and die.*

*I will not die until my mission is accomplished. I will not let the Stalker find me until I've done what I didn't get a chance to do when death came the first time.*

*I will not falter. I will not break. I will not give in to the Thing*

*Behind My Back. At least now, I know who it is. I know its name: Satan.*

It is one of the most common questions that people ask when bad things happen in their lives.

"Why me? What did I do to deserve this? Why is this happening to me?"

I've always been taught that things happen for a reason. I believe that there is a God that is looking out for us. He doesn't do things to us down here simply because He's bored. He's got a plan for each one of us and the things that happen to us during our lives are all done with purpose.

In my simple mind, I thought, *well, if everything happens for a reason. Then I must have been given this disease for a reason.* So I started trying to think of why. Why did this happen to me and not to someone else? Did I do something wrong?

When it first happened to me, I was completely in the dark. I had no idea what I was getting into. The why of the whole thing was the farthest thing in my mind, because I didn't fully understand what was happening. What exactly was this disease called Diabetes? How was it going to affect my everyday life?

The "why" kept escaping me, and I finally came to realize that maybe it wasn't the "why" that I was really after, but the "who." I can tell you from personal experience that it is very tempting to see yourself as someone infected with an incurable disease and think, *thanks a lot God. I can't believe you would do this to me.* It is completely wrong for us to blame God for troubles that happen in our lives. We are told that God allows us to go through things for a reason, but just like Job in the Old Testament, although God allowed for these things to happen to Job, it was Satan who was actually doing the things. God is a loving God who honestly hates to see His creation suffer, but He knows that by allowing us to experience and go through trials we can be made stronger. I knew that God was not to blame and that helped me to deal with what was happening much better than before.

2/12/2002
Dear Journal,

The reason for yesterday's entry was that I had just watched a movie about a kid who had a serious disease and who lived in a hospital with only terminally ill patients.

It made me wonder how someone could live with something like that and still live a normal, productive life. Then I realized that that's exactly what I do. Even though I have something that I can't take away, I try to make the best of it and enjoy life. I don't really need a reason. I don't need to know why. I just have to keep getting up in the morning and pushing myself forward.

Life goes on.

I was once told, "life is not what happens to us, but how we react to it when it does."

# Chapter 10
# Some Didn't Understand

*4/22/2002*
*Dear Journal,*

*I believe that people make fun of me because they are weak, or they simply don't know any better.*

*You know what? I'm not perfect. I'm not better than anyone else. But I'm not trash. I'm not dirt. I'm not lower than the next guy. It's true, I'm cursed. My memory no longer holds onto the days when my life was...normal. My mind used to be where I would escape to when my life was too much to take, but now there's nothing left. When it first happened to me my mind used to torment me with images and thoughts of me after I had been healed. It would haunt my dreams. Now, there's only silence; it has become bored with me.*

*I admit, whether by fault of my curse or by simply my own natural personality, I simply refuse to be like everybody else. I refuse to look, think, act, and talk like the world thinks I should! And then when, after silently taking all of the trash, I let others know that I hurt. That hey! Guess what? When people make you feel like a pitiful freak, it hurts! They tell me that I should just let it slide off of my back and pretend that that stupid comment didn't just come hurtling at me like a poisonous dart!*

*Why am I the one that has to take all of the name-calling and the insults and the teasing? No one understands what goes on inside of a mind that has been poisoned for seven long years! No one understands, and for the most part, they think that if my brain handles things differently than the rest of the dead fish that are content to just go with the flow, there is obviously something wrong with me.*

The world is full of ignorant people that really don't care how a remark is going to make someone else feel. Some do care, but most don't.

If someone were to slip on the iron shackles of my life and walk in them for a week, just one week, they would never again dare to make fun of the unsung hero who doesn't have to merely bear this burden day in and day out, but he has to do it alone! Completely alone, because no one does – or even cares to try to – understand the degree of punishment that goes through my mind every minute. I'm living something that some only see in their nightmares. But I can't ask for help, I can't let anyone that I'm hurting. "Deal with it." "You have twenty minutes to completely forget that you were handed a bombshell." "Get over it."

Mom tries to understand and she tries to help. And in her own motherly way, she does. Most of the time, all she has to do is smile and hug me, without caring about anything else at the moment. She is what is keeping me going, but she is wrong about one thing –

Heroes aren't supposed to cry.

I can only hold on to so much for so long, and then it's going to pour out. Afterwards, I'll simply put my mask on again and face the world, slowly bottling it up again until, after awhile, something else tips the scales. So it's been since I was cursed and so it will be until the curse is lifted.

By God's mercy, it will be lifted!

I ask that you not view me as some bitter, hardened, little boy with a chip on both shoulders. Understand that the feelings that I expressed within the confines of my journal were put there because I felt that they would be dangerous and destructive in the real world. To actually verbalize how I was feeling after situations such as this would not only fail to solve the problem, but would only continue to fuel it. For me, to write something down was to release those feelings from myself harmlessly and quietly.

I know that this is going to be really hard to believe, but I've never been the most popular person around. I know, it's shocking. For my age, I've almost always been the smallest, the skinniest, and the least likely to actually get that ball through the basket.

When it came to sports, I was typically the last kid to be picked for teams. That was just the way life was. Then I got Diabetes and everything changed. They got worse.

There are only a certain amount of insults and names that can be used for a short, skinny kid. But oh! You get a short, skinny *Diabetic* kid and you've got yourself some golden opportunities to make someone feel like the worst thing to ever set foot on the planet. If you run out of names, just push him around; get tired of waiting for him to get back up? You can just make sure and remind him about all of the food that he can't eat. His crushed expression not entertainment enough? Then (worst of all) be sure to let him know just how horrible it must be to have to live with Diabetes, how horrible it must be to be him.

The possibilities were endless and yet I had reached my limit.

I had just reached the seven-year mark two months earlier. The insults from the last seven years were still being stored in some broom closet in my brain. Every time I was hurt by some thoughtless remark, I pretended to ignore it and simply threw it back into that closet along with all the others. As you can imagine, after seven years that closet was beginning to bulge. The door was splintered from the pressure of its contents. All it needed was one more instance stuffed in there and it would finally explode.

That instance came the day of this journal entry. It really wasn't that big of a deal. I've had worse. It really shouldn't have wounded me as badly as it did, but it hit me between the kinks of my armor and pierced me deeply.

My family knew it too. It really shouldn't have hurt me like it did, but the closet door in my mind exploded in a million pieces of splintered wood and the pain hit me harder than I have ever been hurt before.

*4/23/2002*
*Dear Journal,*

*After so long of simply keeping my pain hidden – pretending that it wasn't there and trying to ignore the seemingly endless flood of emotions that I was trying to keep inside – I finally broke down.*

*I was hurt yesterday by comments that someone made to me. They weren't said out of hate or of spite; they were said out of ignorance. He simply didn't know better. It shouldn't have affected me. I've taken harder hits than this before without even flinching, but it was just enough that – when piled on top of all of the other feelings – it spilled over.*

*Thankfully, my parents do understand. No, they don't know to what degree that I suffer, but they want to. They truly want to. Mom held on to me tight as – for the first time in years – I was able to cry. Years ago, I thought that I had become toughened up enough to the point that, even if I tried to, I could not be affected so much by my curse that I would ever show it or express it to anyone else.*

> *I thought that heroes weren't supposed to cry, but even Jesus shed tears.*

*I was wrong. I thought that heroes weren't supposed to cry, but even Jesus shed tears. I thought that if no one completely understood my plight, then no one cared. I know now that at least my parents try, which is really all that I need. Without them, I would simply die.*

*Dad felt bad that he hadn't been caring for me and helping me with my pain like he said he should have. I didn't agree, but he promised to work harder and to do all that he could to help me. That meant the world to me. He and Mom have always been caring for me. They were there when it happened, they were there with me when I came face to face with death, and they are with me now. Thank God for that!*

What can I possibly say about my family? There is no way that I can ever hope to describe the worth of my family. I'm not even sure that an entire book on the subject would do them any sort of justice. No, not even close.

For everyone out there who simply can't relate to the relationship that I have been blessed with in my family, I am sincerely sorry for you. I know that there is no way on earth that I would have been able to overcome the struggles and trials that I have experienced without the help, support, and love that my family gives me everyday. Truthfully, I don't know if they fully understand the impact that they have had on my life.

While other couples could have easily fallen apart under the pressure and stress of having a child with a disease that would eventually claim his life, they have stuck with it. They not only stuck with it, but they succeeded in making our family better for it.

To the unsung heroes that are my parents, I will forever glorify God that He thought me worthy enough to have such people to help me in my walk of life.

If you have been blessed with parents like mine, thank God every day for them. If you haven't, know that God is to all of us the ultimate Father, and He will never let you down.

> *I have never entertained the idea of giving up the fight willingly.*

I have heard stories of Diabetics that have lost all hope of life. They feel that they have struggled too long and too hard and have come to the end of their rope. I have talked to some that have truthfully considered ending their battle and giving up. As frightening as my battle with this disease has been (I have looked death in the face) I have *never* entertained the idea of giving up the fight willingly. My resolve is not there because of merely my own determination or some inner strength of mine. That resolve developed over time because of the family that has stood beside with me and held me up when I no longer had strength to stand on my own.

I speak of a mask that I wore to cover up my emotions. I am amazed at how quickly my mask developed. When I was first hit with the news that my body's cells were attacking their own and that I now had Diabetes, most of the crying that I did was done in the dark when no one was around. I felt that no one could know the pain that I was feeling. I had become upset that no one knew the degree that I hurt, but the truth was that I had always wanted it that way. No one was to know about my pain. I learned early on that if I showed my pain to my mother, it hurt her as well. To keep her from hurting, I had to pretend that I wasn't actually hurting.

On that day, one little remark lit the fire and I blew up. I blew up, and then I went into my room and broke down. After allowing me to lick my wounds long enough in the solitude of my room, Mom finally came in. At first, I didn't want to talk to her. I didn't want her to pull those arrows out, but she did anyway. I only spoke a few sentences to her and then I wept in her arms. I was seventeen years old, crying in my mother's arms.

There were times that I had tried to cry years before, but I couldn't. I had hardened myself to the point that even when I wanted to, I was unable. I would not allow the tears to come. They were held prisoner, as was I.

I don't remember ever crying so hard. I cried about the insult that had occurred that day, but I also cried for that scared ten-year-old boy sitting in that doctor's office. I cried for that delirious young man who was two hours from death. I cried for my mother's pain. I cried for all of the pain that my curse had brought to me. I shook and sobbed. My body ached from crying, but slowly, something inside of me changed. The ache in my spirit was no longer there.

A little while after Mom had left me alone, Dad came in. He had heard about what had happened that day, and had bought me some sugar-free ice cream (one of my favorite desserts) to cheer me up. He apologized for not helping me like he thought he should have. He wanted to take the pain away from me, but truthfully, all I needed was simply for someone to walk next to me; and that's exactly what he had done. I thanked him, hugged him and silently thanked God for him.

I was again left to my own thoughts. It was then that something wonderful happened. After I had taken it off, the mask that had become my hiding place remained on the floor. It was no longer a matter of taking the mask off long enough to let my feelings escape and then putting it back on, content to fool the world (and myself) into thinking that I was unbreakable. Unless I wanted to continue the painful cycle of hiding and ignoring my feelings, the mask had to stay off. It did.

The face that I now see in the mirror is my own. It's an honest face. When I look at it, it's apparent that it has seen its share of battles, but I can also see the victories. Nothing is left hidden behind the eyes.

The truth is that, yes, some people do not understand what it means to live with this disease. Before that day in February when I was ten years old, I had no idea. I had never even heard of the disease, let alone considered the daily battles that those with it must endure.

If this book does nothing else for you, I would pray that it allows you to see us Diabetics in a different light. We are more than people with some disease. We are more than just a statistic. We are more than our disease. *Never define us by our disease.*

Some people do not understand. Do not make the mistake of being one of them.

# Chapter 11
# I Will Not Break

*2/5/1999*
*Dear God,*

*I will not break. I will not give in. With Your help I will stand fast...I will not break.*

This one entry defines me. It is my soul refusing to give up. It is an open rebellion against the forces that try to bring me down.

It is my request to my God to help me, because no matter the level of my own resolve, I know that I can never do it alone. I know that He listens. I know that He can bring me the encouragement and strength that I ask for. He already has. He's given me family, He's given me friends, and He's given me a faith in something better than myself.

We live in a world where comfort is very important. We wear clothes so that we can be comfortable as we go about our lives. We buy soft pillows and mattresses so that even when we're not doing anything at all, we can be comfortable. We don't like to be uncomfortable. It's painful, it's irritating, and it's a serious inconvenience. We feel that if it hurts then it must be a bad thing. We shouldn't be allowed to hurt, and yet what we fail to realize is that pain is a part of life. I've had my share. I believe that everyone who reads this book has the right to say the same. Since we've all experienced it, the question that we should ask ourselves is: when it happened, what did we do? When things became uncomfortable, how did we react? Did we react at all? Did we allow that pain to rule us? Did we allow ourselves to be broken?

God uses these uncomfortable situations to mold us into the kind of person that He knows that we ought to be. If we were never allowed to experience some form of discomfort every now and then, we would never recognize nor fully appreciate the comfort when it arrived. We would take it for granted, as many already do.

I think that the idea of bravery, of standing fast, has been diluted by what Hollywood has been feeding us throughout the years. They tell us that bravery is wielding a weapon and saving the world. They exemplify it with stories of men that stood against entire nations and made memorable speeches just before they galloped out into a sea of enemies. They tell us that bravery is so blatantly apparent that you would have to be blind not to notice one who possessed it. They make us believe that only the strong and handsome people are the brave ones.

*The first few years of my disease were terrible, mainly because I chose to make them that way.*

I've got news for Hollywood: My Diabetic friends Nathan and Diana are brave. Neither of them have ever saved the world from aliens or rescued a child from a burning building, but they have overcome things while living with their disease that some of us can't even imagine. They have witnessed and experienced things that most people are afraid to even talk about. The fear of death has a truer sense of presence in their lives than most people and yet these two people are able to live with a hope, happiness, and an anticipation of the future. These two, along with every Diabetic alive today, are some of the bravest unsung heroes of our time.

I have always been a rather stubborn person. I see things in black and white; right and wrong; true and false. Through my own experience, I have come to realize that although a stubborn nature usually results in trouble, there is a part of me that is thankful to God for blessing me with such a personality trait. The black and white of my disease is this: if I bow under the pressure of my trial, I will allow myself to be consumed by depression and disappointment. To throw in the towel would be to condemn myself to a far worse fate than a mere physical disease. I have recognized the black and white of my situation and my stubborn nature will never allow me to give up. Thank God.

As a message to my fellow sufferers, memorize that entry

written above. Whether you believe in God or not, if you read that passage and firmly resolve within yourself to do exactly and only what you have just read, if you speak those words in your mind, truly believe them, and (most importantly) act according to that belief, you will become that soldier that we all want to be on the inside.

Understand that I'm not here to offer medical advice. I'm not here to condemn nor condone the choices of anyone. So why write this? What is the purpose of this book?

I am amazed at the gradual changes in my attitude as I read through my journal entries. The first few years of my disease were terrible, mainly because I chose to make them that way. I viewed my disease as a curse, as a burden that had been unjustly placed upon me. I figured that any hope of a normal life was gone. During those first few years I was overcome with sadness. I would cry myself to sleep at night and pray earnestly for no one but myself.

A few years went by and death visited me. My life perspective changed, and rightly so. I realized that it wasn't always going to be about me. The well being of others was more important that my own personal comfort. However, I still resented the disease and the baggage that came with it. I was in my teenage years and had to deal with my ever immature and insensitive peers that enjoyed bringing me down. I built for myself a mask that I would put on whenever I would hurt. I was not protecting myself, but hiding myself from those who really cared about me.

I continued using the mask for years. I stored the insults and ridicule away in the closest of my mind. This was dangerous, because when the door could no longer withstand the pressure of its contents, it would crash open. My anger would burst forth, wounding countless others in its wake. There finally came a moment after such an emotional devastation, that I made an important decision. I had believed in the world's idea of a hero: someone who shows no fear, no pain, and no emotion. I finally realized that I was not out to become a worldly hero, but a godly one. The mask came off, and I left it on the floor.

Then I went through the typical phase of asking God why. Why did He allow this to happen? Why did He choose me? What did I ever do to deserve this? Everyone does this at some point in their lives; they question their Creator. I never actually questioned His existence or His providence, but simply His purpose. After years of wrestling with these questions, He made me understand that He had allowed me to have it because He knew that I would be able to handle it. While it seemed overwhelming at first, He knew that in time I would be able to overcome. It was given to me, and not to the members of my family, and that was a tremendous blessing.

At long last, I came to realize the reason that I was diagnosed with Diabetes. I was given it to learn things that I never would have learned any other way.

I learned that other people come first. There are other people that are in more need of healing than you are. Life isn't about living for yourself. It's about looking out for others, because in turn, they will look out for you.

I learned that family is a gift from God. There is a reason that God did not choose to allow man to raise himself. He gave us family, whether truly blood related or simply committed individuals, to lean on in times of troubles and we should thank God for them everyday.

I learned that being a true hero means more than simply appearing brave. Heroes are more than allowed to feel, they are required to.

I learned that everything is done for a reason. God has a plan for each of us, and while it's very likely we may not fully comprehend His plan, we simply need to trust Him.

I have told my story and explained the choices that we made concerning my disease because it is my hope that somehow this book may touch your life in some positive way.

I wrote this book for myself. I have come a long way since February 28, 1995. I have matured from the scared, skinny, little boy sitting in the doctor's office, into a Diabetic that is no longer afraid. I am no longer afraid of the needle pricks, I am no longer afraid of the insults that I have and will continue to receive. Most importantly, I am no longer afraid of death. Diabetes motivated me to develop an unshakable resolve that no force on earth will ever tear down: my faith.

I wrote this book for the millions of Diabetics like me. I have shared my story with you as a way to continue what I once prayed to God for: the opportunity to heal others. The bottom line is this...

Everyone will experience unchangeable hardships, ours just happens to be a disease. Simply remember,

- We are *not* defined by our disease.
- It will only break us if we allow it.
- Life changing events are occurring all of the time. Don't resent them. Learn from them.

This book was written to the rest of the world. I pray that in telling my story, I have been successful in putting a face on what once may have been unknown to you. More than simply supplying recognition to this disease is my hope of challenging you to look at Diabetes in a different light. I pray that you can now view it with more understanding and with the well-deserved respect for the millions of heroes that fight the battle of Diabetes everyday. The question is never how much information you have gathered, but what you plan to do with that information now that you have it.

Finally, this book was written for my mother, Linda Dehut. If this book pleases none but her, the words would not have been ill spent. I doubt that even she fully understands all that she has done for me. She kept me from allowing this disease to consume me. She took my hand and pulled me from the monster's clutches those many times that it came so close to devouring me. I honestly believe that the reason death came for me and left without his quarry was because a mother loved her son too much.

She is the reason that I finally chose to lay aside my own pain, fear, and disappointment, don my suit of armor and fight for something. I have courage now, but she has always possessed it. I have strength now, but it is only what has been lent to me from her. I am a soldier, but no mere soldier at that. I am hers. I fight for her, and there can be no more a worthy cause.

My name is Craig Daniel Dehut, and I have Diabetes.

*2/28/2003*
*Dear Journal,*

*The battle rages on. This soldier has seen his share of pain, suffering, and hopelessness. This soldier has seen his share of healing, hope, and victory.*

*No one even thinks about it anymore...sooner or later, this monster will claim my life. It will...but not yet.*

*I haven't changed the world yet.*

*And I would love to see this disease just try and stop me.*

## THE END

## ABOUT THE AUTHOR

Craig Daniel Dehut was diagnosed with Type 1 Juvenile Diabetes at the age of ten. With the help and support of his family and friends, he has learned to take care of himself and to enjoy life as a healthy, creative Christian.

Craig was homeschooled and graduated from the Art Institute of Atlanta in 2007 with a Fine Arts degree in Video Production. His goal is to continue to use the talents that he has been given in the service of God and others.

**The Lion is the Lamb (Andrew Roberts)**

Study of the King of Kings, His glorious kingdom, & promised return

**When Opportunity Knocks (Matthew Allen)**

Lessons on how to meet the JW's/Mormons who knock on your door

**Reveal In Me... (Jeanne Sullivan)**

A ladies study on finding and developing one's own talents

**I Will NOT Be Lukewarm, Ppt/Teacher's Manual (Dana Burk)**

A ladies study on defeating mediocrity

**The Gospel of John (Cassondra Givans)**

A study for women, by a woman, on this letter of John

**Sisters at War (Cassondra Givans)**

Breaking the generation gap between sisters in Christ

**Will You Wipe My Tears? (Joyce Jamerson)**

Resources to teach us how to help others through sorrow

**Bridges or Barriers, w/Manual (Cindy DeBerry/Angie Kmitta)**

Study encouraging harmony with younger/older sisters-in-Christ

**Learning to Sing at Midnight (Joanne Beckley)**

A study book about spiritual growth benefiting women of all ages

**Transitions, with Ppt/Teacher's Manual (Ken Weliever)**

A relevant life study for this changing age group

**Snapshots: Defining Moments in a Girl's Life (Nicole Sardinas)**

How to make godly decisions when it really matters

**The Path of Peace (Cassondra Givans)**

Relevant and important topics of study for teens

**The Purity Pursuit (Andrew Roberts)**

Helping teens achieve purity in all aspects of life

**Paul's Letter to the Romans (Matthew Allen)**

Putting righteousness by faith on an understandable level

**AUTISM, In the Eye of the Hurricane (Juli Liske)**

A family's journey from the shock of an autistic diagnosis to victory

**For However Brief a Time (Warren Berkley)**

A son's human interest tales of his father in a time now gone by

**Family Bible Study Series (Ken Weliever)**

A series of 16 quarters of Bible class curriculum ideas

www.ingramcontent.com/pod-product-compliance
Lightning Source LLC
Chambersburg PA
CBHW030825060726
47590CB00004B/1397